# GENTLE YOGA

## MULTIPLE SCLEROSIS

Featuring Contributions By

# LAURIE SANFORD

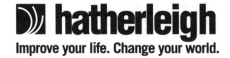

**hatherleigh**

Improve your life. Change your world.

Gentle Yoga for Multiple Sclerosis

Text copyright © 2012 Hatherleigh Press

Hatherleigh Press is committed to preserving and protecting the natural resources of the Earth. Environmentally responsible and sustainable practices are embraced within the company's mission statement. Hatherleigh Press is a member of the Publishers Earth Alliance, committed to preserving and protecting the natural resources of the planet while developing a sustainable business model for the book publishing industry.

This book was edited and designed in the village of Hobart, New York. Hobart is a community that has embraced books and publishing as a component of its livelihood. There are several unique bookstores in the village. For more information, please visit www.hobartbookvillage.com.

Library of Congress Cataloging-in-Publication Data is available.
ISBN: 978-1-57826-370-7

Disclaimer
Consult your physician before beginning any exercise program. The author and publisher of this book and workout disclaim any liability, personal or professional, resulting from the misapplication of any of the following procedures described in this publication.

All Hatherleigh Press titles are available for bulk purchase, special promotions, and premiums. For information about reselling and special purchase opportunities, please call 1-800-528-2550 and ask for the Special Sales Manager.

Cover Design by Heather Daugherty
Interior Design by Heather White
Photography by Catarina Astrom

10 9 8 7 6 5 4 3 2 1

Printed in the United States

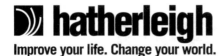

Improve your life. Change your world.

www.hatherleighpress.com

# TABLE OF CONTENTS

# ACKNOWLEDGMENTS

Hatherleigh Press would like to extend a special thank you to Jo Brielyn—without your hard work and dedication this book would not have been possible.

# CHAPTER 1

## WHAT IS MULTIPLE SCLEROSIS?

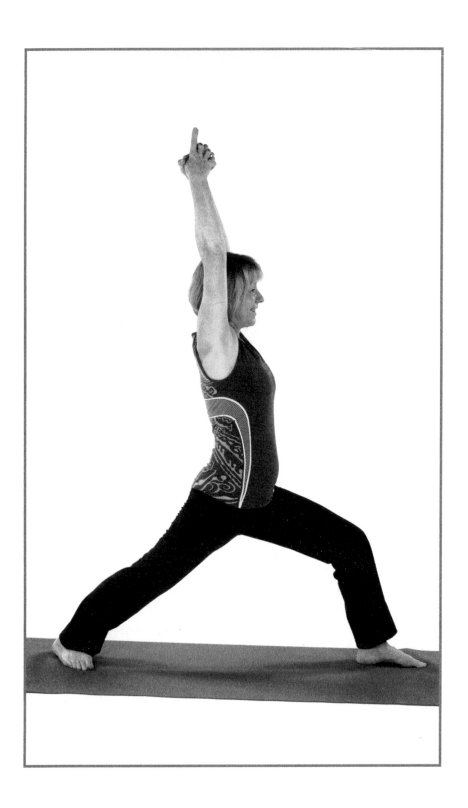

Multiple sclerosis (MS) is a chronic disease that affects the *central nervous system (CNS)* of the body, the system that consists of the brain, spinal cord, and optic nerves. Multiple sclerosis is believed to be an autoimmune disease, which means that the body is attacked by its own immune system. When multiple sclerosis is present, the white blood cells that would normally fight infection or illness instead attack and destroy the soft, fatty tissue (*myelin*) that surrounds the nerves in the spinal cord and brain. Inflammation in the central nervous system occurs when the myelin is attacked by the immune system. This process is known as *demyelination*. The myelin that breaks down during demyelination is replaced by thick scar tissue known as *plaques*. With less myelin to serve as a shield and insulator and more scar tissue to divert the path, nerve impulses sent from the brain to the rest of the body become jumbled, misdirected, or blocked.

The name "multiple sclerosis" originates from the presence of those plaques. "Multiple" refers to the many plaques present and "sclerosis" means scars. So the literal meaning of the disease's name is multiple scars.

Although each person will experience a unique combination of symptoms, there are a number of distinct patterns that may occur with multiple sclerosis. In 1996, the United States National Multiple Sclerosis Society standardized four subtypes of multiple sclerosis:

*Relapsing-Remitting Multiple Sclerosis:* There are unpredictable relapses or attacks with this form of multiple sclerosis during which new symptoms may surface or existing symptoms can become more severe. The relapse may last for days or months and the individual then experiences a partial or total remission (recovery). The disease may remain inactive for several months or years. This is the most common pattern found as approximately 85 percent of people with multiple sclerosis are initially diagnosed with relapsing-remitting MS.

*Primary Progressive Multiple Sclerosis:* Primary progressive MS makes up about 10 percent of the diagnosed cases. It is generally distinguished by slowly developing and steadily worsening symptoms, but a lack of distinct attacks. Disabilities and symptoms associated with this MS pattern may stabilize at some point or can continue for several months or years.

*Secondary Progressive Multiple Sclerosis:* Some patients who are initially diagnosed with relapsing-remitting MS may experience a progressive disability later in the course of the disease. This is known as secondary progressive MS and often includes overlapping relapses with no distinct remission periods.

*Progressive Relapsing Multiple Sclerosis:* A small number of multiple sclerosis patients may experience a steady decline and overlapping attacks without remissions. They may or may not have some form of recovery after the relapses. This is the least common category and encompasses only about 5 percent of multiple sclerosis patients.

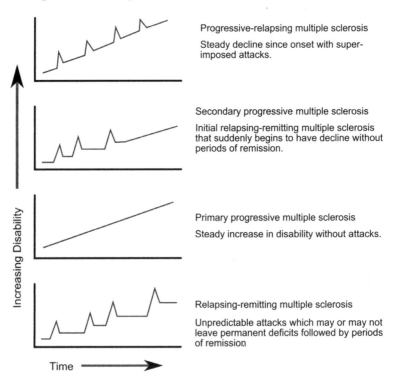

Progressive-relapsing multiple sclerosis

Steady decline since onset with super-imposed attacks.

Secondary progressive multiple sclerosis

Initial relapsing-remitting multiple sclerosis that suddenly begins to have decline without periods of remission.

Primary progressive multiple sclerosis

Steady increase in disability without attacks.

Relapsing-remitting multiple sclerosis

Unpredictable attacks which may or may not leave permanent deficits followed by periods of remission

Increasing Disability

Time

## Causes of Multiple Sclerosis

There are currently over 2.5 million people who have been diagnosed with multiple sclerosis. In the United States alone, there are about 400,000 people living with MS and over 200 more people are diagnosed each week. The Multiple Sclerosis Association of America reports that approximately 10,000 to 15,000 new cases of multiple sclerosis are diagnosed every year in the United States.

The disease is most commonly found in people between the ages of 20 and 40 years old, but can affect people of any age. Of those cases reported, more women than men are affected by multiple sclerosis. Individuals of Caucasian descent also seem to be more likely to develop the disease.

Since the nerves in any part of the brain or spinal cord can be damaged by multiple sclerosis, MS patients may experience symptoms in various parts of the body. While those symptoms can range from mild to severe, there is absolutely no evidence to suggest that multiple sclerosis is in any way contagious or infectious. Although the symptoms of the disease can certainly be life-altering, it is rare for multiple sclerosis to progress to a terminal stage. While severe cases can shorten one's life span, the majority of individuals who have MS live close to normal life expectancy.

## Risk Factors for Multiple Sclerosis

There are many factors that lead to MS, some that can be changed and others that cannot. Awareness of these risk factors is important to the prevention, early diagnosis, and treatment of multiple sclerosis.

**Common fixed risk factors for multiple sclerosis include:**

*Age:* Multiple sclerosis can occur in people of any age, but it most often affects people between the ages of 20 and 40 years old. Although not impossible, MS can, in rare cases, develop before the age of 15 or after 60.

*Gender:* While anyone can develop the disease, women are two to three times more likely to develop multiple sclerosis than men. However, there is some research which indicates that men are often more disabled by MS than women.

*Genetics:* Multiple Sclerosis is not directly inherited, but scientists have been able to identify that there are genetic factors that affect susceptibility and contribute to a higher risk of developing the disease. If a parent or sibling has the disease, a person has a 1 to 3 percent chance of developing multiple sclerosis. The general population has only one-tenth of 1 percent risk.

*Race:* Statistics show that people who are Caucasian, especially those with family origins in northern Europe, are at the highest risk of developing MS. The lowest risk for multiple sclerosis seems to be for individuals of Native American, African, and Asian descent.

*Having other diseases that affect immunity:* People who have other diseases like thyroid disease, type 1 diabetes, or inflammatory bowel disease have a slightly higher risk of developing multiple sclerosis.

*Having certain infections:* There are a variety of viral and bacterial infections that have been linked to MS patients. Scientists are currently conducting research on many of the infections in question to determine if they play a role or how big a part they play in the development of multiple sclerosis. One that is causing the greatest concern is the connection between patients who develop multiple sclerosis and have also had the Epstein-Barr virus—the virus that causes infectious mononucleosis.

*Living in areas with temperate climates and increased latitude:* The disease is more prevalent in people who live in northern United States, southern Canada, Europe, New Zealand, and southeastern Australia. There appears to be an increased risk of developing MS associated with the increase in latitude. It is also less prevalent in tropical and subtropical regions. Children who move from an area with one risk level to another tend to conform to the risk level associated with the new area. However, for adults and people past puberty, the risk level related to their first home seems to be retained.

**Modifiable risk factors for multiple sclerosis include:**

*History of smoking cigarettes:* In addition to the harmful effects cigarettes that have on the heart and lungs, studies show there is evidence that smoking may increase the risk of developing MS.

*Poor nutrition:* The lack of a well-balanced diet and deficiencies in important nutrients like vitamin D make individuals more prone to developing multiple sclerosis and less able to deal with its symptoms.

**You can contact these national organizations to learn more about multiple sclerosis, ask specific questions, or receive additional data related to the disease:**

MS Awareness Foundation
Toll-free phone number: (888) 336-6723 (MSAF)
Website: www.msawareness.org
Email: info@msawareness.org

Multiple Sclerosis Association of America
Toll-free phone number: (800) 532-7667
Website: www.msaa.com
Email: MSquestions@msassociation.org

Multiple Sclerosis Foundation
Toll-free phone number: (800) 225-6495
For the Program Services Assistance MS Helpline, call toll-free: (888) MSFOCUS
Website: www.msfacts.org
Email: support@msfocus.org

Multiple Sclerosis International Federation
Phone number: +44 (0) 20 7620 1911
Website: www.msif.org
Email: info@msif.org

National Multiple Sclerosis Society
Toll-free phone number: (800) 344-4867
Website: www.nationalmssociety.org
To request additional information:
www.nationalmssociety.org/ContactUs.aspx

## Symptoms and Diagnosis of Multiple Sclerosis

Symptoms of multiple sclerosis vary greatly because the location and severity of each MS attack is different. Episodes associated with the disease may last for days, weeks, or even months. Symptoms may stop or may not be as severe when the individual is experiencing a remission from a multiple sclerosis episode. The next relapse may or may not include the same symptoms as the one prior to it.

The location, size, and amount of the plaques caused by demyelination may determine the symptoms and their severity. Often, though, there may be no significant increase in symptoms even while disease activity is continuing to take place within the central nervous system. The specific signs associated with multiple sclerosis and their severity also vary greatly from person to person.

Plaques found in the cerebrum and cerebellum will trigger symptoms such as balance and coordination problems, tremors, and issues with speech. If plaques are located in the sensory nerve tract, the patient may experience issues such as burning, prickly feelings, numbness, and other altered sensations. Plaques around the motor nerve tracts will influence symptoms like bladder and bowel complications, muscle weakness, spasticity, vision problems, and paralysis.

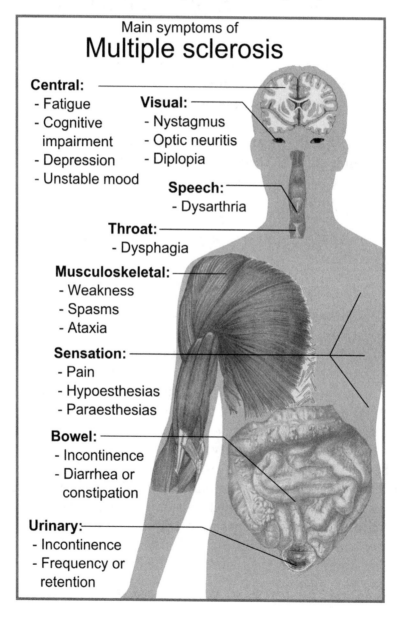

Main symptoms of
# Multiple sclerosis

**Central:**
- Fatigue
- Cognitive impairment
- Depression
- Unstable mood

**Visual:**
- Nystagmus
- Optic neuritis
- Diplopia

**Speech:**
- Dysarthria

**Throat:**
- Dysphagia

**Musculoskeletal:**
- Weakness
- Spasms
- Ataxia

**Sensation:**
- Pain
- Hypoesthesias
- Paraesthesias

**Bowel:**
- Incontinence
- Diarrhea or constipation

**Urinary:**
- Incontinence
- Frequency or retention

The most common early symptoms of multiple sclerosis include a loss of balance, weakness in the limbs, tingling and numbness, and blurred or doubled vision. Below is a more comprehensive list of the signs and symptoms that people with multiple sclerosis may experience.

**Possible symptoms of multiple sclerosis include:**

*Visual Symptoms:*
• Optic Neuritis: Optic neuritis occurs in about 55 percent of multiple sclerosis patients. It causes pain and blurring or graying of vision, generally in one eye at a time.
• Double vision (also known as *diplopia*)
• Jerky or rapid eye movements (called *nystagmus*)
• Flashing lights in response to sounds or eye movement
• Lack of coordination between the two eyes
• Eye discomfort
• Total loss of sight: Blindness associated with the disease is rare and usually only occurs in the most severe cases of multiple sclerosis

*Motor Symptoms:*
• Muscle weakness, most commonly in the arms and legs
• Spasticity: Spasticity is the loss of muscle tone in the limbs that results in pain and stiffness and usually makes it difficult to move freely. This symptom occurs in the initial MS attack for about 40 percent of people and is later present in over 60 percent of individuals with more progressive stages of the disease. Depending on the severity, spasticity can affect the individual's mobility and ability to walk unassisted.
• Muscle spasms and cramps
• Tremors: Tremors associated with MS generally include shaking or trembling of the limbs or head. Up to 50 percent of multiple sclerosis patients report problems with tremors and other shaky movements.
• Tics and involuntary twitches in the muscles
• Restless leg syndrome

- Difficulty swallowing or chewing (also called *dysphagia*)
- Problems with posture
- Paralysis: This may vary from partial, nearly all, or total paralysis.

*Sensory Symptoms:*
- Paraesthesia: Numbness, tingling, and unusual sensations may occur in any area of the body.
- Facial pain
- Electric shocks, especially involving movement of the head
- Burning and itching sensations
- Anaesthesia: Total numbness and loss of sensation can occur in extreme cases.

*Coordination and Balance Symptoms:*
- Ataxia: Many people with multiple sclerosis suffer from ataxia, which is a loss of coordination that makes walking unstable.
- Vertigo: Some individuals with multiple sclerosis may experience dizziness, nausea and vomiting along with balance issues.
- Inability or impaired ability to rapidly change movements (such as the movements required to dance or move to a rhythm)
- Dysmetria: Dysmetria is a coordination issue that causes the individual to under- or over-shoot movements with the limbs or eyes. This symptom can make picking up objects difficult for the patient.
- Loss of balance

*Cognitive Symptoms:*
- Dementia
- Issues with short-term and long-term memory: Problems with memory affect about two-thirds of all multiple sclerosis patients to some degree.
- Forgetfulness
- Moods swings

• Anxiety
• Depression: Depression is a common reaction to diagnosis of many illnesses, and MS is no exception. However, it is important to be aware that fatigue and lethargy that are often symptoms of multiple sclerosis can sometimes be mistaken for depression.
• Bipolar disorder
• Slurred speech, slowing of speech, and trouble recalling words
• Difficulty with speech comprehension
• Decreased attention span

*Other Symptoms:*
• Fatigue: Fatigue is one of the most common symptoms of MS. The fatigue is unpredictable and not proportionate to the amount of physical activity the person has done. Multiple sclerosis patients often complain of being tired even after having a full night's sleep.
• Lethargy
• Acid reflux
• Impaired sense of smell and taste
• Sleeping disorders
• Sexual dysfunctions: Over 90 percent of men and 70 percent of women report changes in their sexual activity after developing MS. Common issues are impotence, decreased sexual drive, impaired sensation, and loss of interest.
• Sensitivity to heat or cold
• Bladder problems and incontinence
• Constipation
• Diarrhea or bowel incontinence

## Common Triggers for Multiple Sclerosis Attacks

Multiple sclerosis symptoms often occur in cycles. You may find that your MS symptoms are minimal one day and increase radically the next. This is generally referred to as an MS attack or relapse. There are some environmental, physical, and emotional factors that may trigger a relapse and increase the pain associated with your disease. By learning how to regulate or make accommodations for these triggers, you may be able to keep your pain levels lower and reduce the frequency and severity of your multiple sclerosis symptoms.

**Factors that can trigger an attack or relapse include:**

• Fever
• Hot baths or heated pools
• Too much exposure to sun
• Stress
• Viral infections (like the flu, common cold, or gastroenteritis)
• Pregnancy (especially postpartum)

## Common Treatments for MS

There is no known cure for multiple sclerosis at this time. There are, however, a variety of therapies that may help slow the progression of the disease. The goal of treatment for multiple sclerosis is to control the symptoms and help patients obtain and maintain a healthy quality of life.

The types of treatment for multiple sclerosis fall into two main categories: symptom management and treatments that modify the amount and severity of relapses and disability. Over the past ten years, there has been significant progress made in both of these areas.

Since 1993, the U.S. Food and Drug Administration (FDA) had approved six different medications used for disease-modifying treatment of multiple sclerosis: Betaseron®, Avonex®, Rebif®, Copaxone®, Tysabri®, and Novantrone®.

**Therapies, alternative treatments, and lifestyle changes that may be helpful include:**

- Physical therapy
- Speech therapy
- Occupational therapy
- Attending support groups
- Installation of assisting devices such as bed lifts, wall bars, and shower chairs
- Making minor safety adjustments in the home to protect against falls
- Use of walkers, motorized scooters, or wheelchairs
- Getting involved with a structured exercise program in the earlier stages of the disease
- Massage
- Acupuncture
- Reflexology
- Meditation
- Practicing yoga and other stress-relieving methods
- Adapting a healthy lifestyle, including adequate rest and good nutrition

## Foods to Include in a Healthy Diet for Multiple Sclerosis Patients

**Some dietary recommendations for people with multiple sclerosis include:**

*Drink plenty of water:* Try to drink about two quarts of water each day and reduce or eliminate your consumption of caffeinated beverages, which dehydrate the body. Drinking water helps fight constipation, which is a common complaint among people with multiple sclerosis. Of course, if you have trouble with bladder incontinence, adjustments may have to be made.

*Eat a fiber-rich diet*: A diet high in fiber should include a variety of whole grains (especially bran, oats, or flax), vegetables, and fruits (particularly prunes).

*Include fish and omega-3 fatty acids:* These are found in oily fish and fish oil supplements. They protect against inflammation and are believed to help with some of the symptoms associated with MS and autoimmune disorders.

There are also some vitamins and nutrients that are especially vital to nerve function and, therefore, will prove beneficial to individuals who have multiple sclerosis. Begin by increasing your intake of vitamin B12, vitamins A and vitamin D in your diet. Below are some natural ways to add these and other important vitamins and nutrients to your diet to boost and maintain your health:

**Natural Sources of Vitamin B12:**
• Liver
• Lean beef
• Clams
• Salmon
• Haddock
• Trout
• Dairy (such as cheese and eggs)

**Natural Sources of Vitamin A:**
• Dairy products (such as milk and eggs)
• Yellow vegetables (summer squash)
• Carrots
• Liver
• Green leafy vegetables (such as kale, spinach, greens, and romaine lettuce)
• Fruits (such as cantaloupe, tomatoes, and apricots)

**Natural Sources of Vitamin D:**
• Sunlight

- Dairy products (such as milk and eggs)
- Tuna
- Liver oils
- Mackerel
- Cod
- Sea bass

**Natural Sources of Calcium:**
- Dairy products (such as milk, cheese, and plain low-fat yogurt)
- Sardines
- Salmon
- Any seafood that contains bones
- Turnip greens
- Spinach
- Kale
- Broccoli
- Nuts (such as almonds, Brazil nuts, and pecans)
- Legumes (such as peas, lentils, and beans)

**Natural Sources of Potassium:**
- Milk
- Green leafy vegetables (such as romaine lettuce, spinach, and Swiss chard)
- Broccoli
- Lentils
- Winter squash
- Fruits (such as tomatoes, cantaloupe, avocado, oranges, and strawberries)
- Snapper
- Halibut
- Scallops
- Soy
- Potatoes (white and sweet varieties)

**Natural Sources of Copper:**
- Vegetables

- Liver
- Legumes
- Nuts
- Seeds
- Beans

**Natural Sources of Magnesium:**
- Brazil nuts
- Seeds (such as sunflower seeds, pumpkin seeds, and sesame seeds)
- Bananas
- Legumes
- Tofu
- Green leafy vegetables (such a spinach, Swiss chard, and kelp)
- Whole grains (such as barley, brown rice, and oats)

## Famous and Notable People with MS

- James Scofield, poet
- Natalie Mandzhavidze, NASA physicist
- Montel Williams, talk show host/actor
- Richard Pryor, comedian and actor
- David Humm, NFL quarterback for the Oakland Raiders
- Lena Horne, actress and singer
- Mary Mullarkey, Colorado State Supreme Court Chief Justice
- Annette Funicello, singer, dancer, and former Mouseketeer
- Betty Cuthbert, Olympic Gold Medalist for sprinting
- Neil Cavuto, lead anchor on Fox News Channel
- Clive Burr, drummer for Iron Maiden
- Adam Riedy, US speed skater
- Bill Bradbury, Secretary of State of Oregon
- Michael Blake, Hollywood screenwriter best known for *Dances with Wolves*
- Sarah P. Gibbs, biologist and winner of the 2003 Gilbert Morgan Smith Medal

## Did You Know?

• More women than men are diagnosed with multiple sclerosis.
• People who live closer to the equator (and are exposed to more sunlight) are less likely to develop MS.
• Multiple sclerosis is the most common progressive and disabling neurological condition found in young adults.
• Multiple sclerosis was first labeled in 1868 by a French neurologist named Jean-Martin Charcot.
• It takes an average of four to five years from the clinical onset of multiple sclerosis until a diagnosis is made by a physician.
• The average age of diagnosis for MS patients is 37 years old.
• The risk among the general population of developing MS is about 1 in 800.
• Around 20 to 40 percent of women with multiple sclerosis will experience a relapse within the first three months after giving birth.
• There is no clear cause or cure for MS.

# CHAPTER 2

## THE BENEFITS OF YOGA

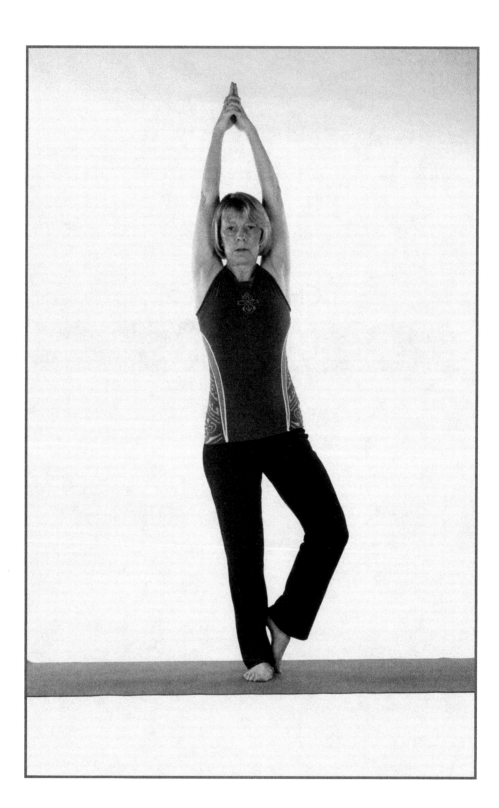

Physical activity is important for people with multiple sclerosis, although some may have difficulty engaging in more strenuous forms of exercise. Yoga is one form of exercise that is now becoming a recognized method of treatment and physical activity for people with MS because it can be adapted and modified to meet the specific needs of each individual.

The poses found in this book have been designed to accommodate various stages of the disease and include variations to help you tailor your yoga practice to your own level of mobility. If you are currently using a wheelchair, you may find the chair variations helpful. However, always be sure to listen to your body and only do poses that feel safe and comfortable for you.

Yoga combines both weight-bearing exercises and muscle-strengthening exercises, making it a wise choice for people with multiple sclerosis. It is also a low-impact form of physical activity, so there is less danger of loss of balance or falls that may accompany more high-impact forms of exercise.

**In addition to being a low-impact and customizable form of exercise, yoga also:**

*Offers relief from pain, stress and anxiety:* Yoga is effective in alleviating pain, and reducing stress and anxiety, which can compromise systems in your body and affect functions like immunity and digestion. Yoga practices such as meditation help the individual focus on something other than what he or she feels. It also allows the entire body to relax and get the rest it needs to replenish itself.

*Strengthens muscles and increases flexibility:* Strong and flexible muscles boost the strength of the bones they surround and offer them added protection. Yoga provides a way to strengthen muscles and build flexibility without making your muscles too bulky. Strengthening your muscles, particularly those in the back and shoulders, also helps improve your posture. Yoga also helps release tension in the muscles, which in turn helps relieve the spasticity common among MS patients.

*Creates balance and coordination*: Yoga is beneficial for individuals who have multiple sclerosis because it improves balance and coordination, which will make you more stable on your feet and help reduce the number of falls you take.

## Yoga and the Mind-Body Connection

Yoga is a mind-body kind of exercise that helps you stay fit and relaxed, and is also beneficial for managing chronic back pain. Since yoga combines movement and conscious breathing exercises, it helps you focus both on what your body is physically doing and what is occurring internally. As the root "yuj" (meaning unity or yoke) implies, yoga is an exercise form that seeks to unify the mind and body. When that union takes place, it brings with it a wealth of therapeutic benefits.

The practice of yoga can be traced back to over 5000 years ago, to a time when monks in India (called *yogi*) secluded themselves and sat for hours in deep meditation in an attempt to create strong, disease-free bodies. While they found the meditation good for the mind, their sore bodies would not allow them to stay in the same position for extended periods. Instead, they had to change positions while still focusing on their meditation. Over time, more structured yoga postures stemmed from these early practices and addressed specific needs in the body as well as the mind.

Today, yoga is used in many therapeutic ways, such as to detoxify, relieve anxiety and depression, realign musculature, strengthen muscles, create flexibility, and manage chronic pain.

*"Yoga teaches us to cure what need not be endured, and endure what cannot be cured." —B.K.S. Iyengar*

**Learn more about yoga and
its benefits on these websites:**

American Yoga Association
www.americanyogaassociation.org

International Association of Yoga Therapists
www.iayt.org

Yoga Journal
www.yogajournal.com

## Stress Relievers: Breathing, Meditation, and Visual Imagery

The manner in which you respond to stress may exacerbate your existing symptoms or induce a multiple sclerosis attack. For instance, stress often prompts more instances of sleep problems, overeating, abuse of alcohol and illicit drugs, and smoking.

### A Breathing Exercise: The Gateway to Daily Meditation

Focusing on the breath is one of the most common and fundamental techniques for accessing the meditative state. Breath is a deep rhythm of the body that connects us intimately with the world around us. Learn these steps, and then practice them as a regular breathing exercise.

Close your eyes, breathe deeply and regularly, and observe your breath as it flows in through the nose and out of the mouth. Give your full attention to the breath as it comes in and goes out. Store your breath in the belly, not the chest, between inhales and exhales. Whenever you find your attention wandering away from your breath, gently pull it back to the rising and falling of the breath via the belly.

Inhale through your nose slowly and deeply, feeling the lower chest and abdomen inflate like a balloon. Hold for five seconds. Exhale deeply, deflating the lower chest and abdomen like an emptying balloon. Hold for five seconds. Do this five times, and then allow your breathing to return to a normal rhythm.

You will begin to feel a change come over your entire body. Gradually you will become less aware of your breathing, but not captured in your stream of consciousness. Consciousness is encouraged on the whole, but we often are too alert and hyper-stimulated via TV, caffeine, and family life, just to name a few. By breathing for five minutes daily, you will become more centered inward. You will just live "in the moment," in your own skin.

## Benefits of a simple breathing exercise throughout the day include:

• Calming
• "Re-centering" one's thoughts
• Increase in oxygenated blood flow, improved efficiency expiring carbon dioxide
• Decreased levels of fatigue later in the day, legs won't feel "heavy"

Increasing oxygenated blood via deep breathing can decrease muscle pains, especially in the postural muscles (back and neck muscles), and help counteract chronic stressors such as sitting or standing in static positions for extended periods of time.

## Deep Breathing

Practice deep breathing as a form of relaxation before bed. Slow, deep breathing is an excellent way to slow the heart rate and contemplate the day's events. Focus on breathing in through the nose and out through the mouth.

## Meditation Tips for Beginners

Yoga offers meditation and controlled breathing techniques that are used effectively to manage the pain associated with your multiple sclerosis and refocus your thoughts. Meditating for only a few minutes each day can help.

## Simple Stress Reliever

Looking for a simple, healthy way to help get through the day? Try breathing exercises—a wonderfully effective way to reduce stress, maintain focus, and feel energized. Exhaling completely is one breathing exercise to try—it can promote deeper breathing and better health.

**Give it a try:** Simply take a deep breath, let it out effortlessly, and then squeeze out a little more. Doing this regularly will help build up the muscles between your ribs, and your exhalations will soon become deeper and longer. Start by practicing this exhalation exercise consciously, and before long it will become a healthy, unconscious habit.

## Here are a few quick tips for meditation beginners:

• Take the time to stretch out first. Loosening muscles and tendons before beginning allows you to sit or lie more comfortably.

• Make it a formal practice by setting aside a specific time and place to devote to your meditation.

• Focus on the breathing. Slowing your breathing helps your mind and body to relax and prepare for meditation.

• Meditate in the morning. It is usually quieter in the morning, and your mind has not yet had the chance to get cluttered. It will also help you work out any kinks in your body from sleeping. And it's always great to start your day with focus!

• Find a time and place to meditate where you will not be disturbed.

• Enlist the help of instructional videos or calming music if they help you relax more.

• Light a candle and use it as a focal point, instead of closing your eyes. Focusing on the light causes you to strengthen your attention.

• Be aware of your body and how it feels in both its normal and relaxed states, and embrace the differences.

• Experiment with different types of meditation and different positions. You won't know which methods work best for you until you try them.

• Have a purpose behind your meditation, such as pain management or feeling more focused on a specific issue you must deal with.

• Push aside any feelings of doubt, frustration, and stress about whether or not you are doing it right. It is counterproductive to your meditation.

• Relax and relish in your mind's incredible ability to focus and care for your body through meditation.

• Remember your meditation and breathing techniques throughout the day. A few well-placed cleansing breaths will do wonders for your mind and body.

**Many of the most commonly recommended yoga poses for multiple sclerosis can be found in this book, including:**

Warm-Up Forward Bend
Warrior I
Warrior II
Warrior III
Downward-Facing Dog
Upward-Facing Dog
Reverse Warrior
Triangle
Tree
Cobra
Plank
Boat
Locust
Child

## Did You Know?

• Yoga has been practiced in America since the late 19th century but only gained popularity around the 1960s.
• Yoga can relieve pain from many chronic conditions.
• According to the Benson-Henry Institute for Mind-Body Medicine (previously the Mind Body Medical Institute at Harvard Medical School), chronic pain patients who practice meditation reduce their physician visits by 36%.
• Yoga can be practiced virtually anywhere. Variations can even be done at your desk or in your car.
• Yoga and diet go hand in hand. There are foods you can eat that will actually increase your brain function and flexibility.
• A man who practices yoga is called a *yogi* or *yogin*. A woman who does is called a *yogini*.

# CHAPTER 3

## SAFETY PRECAUTIONS

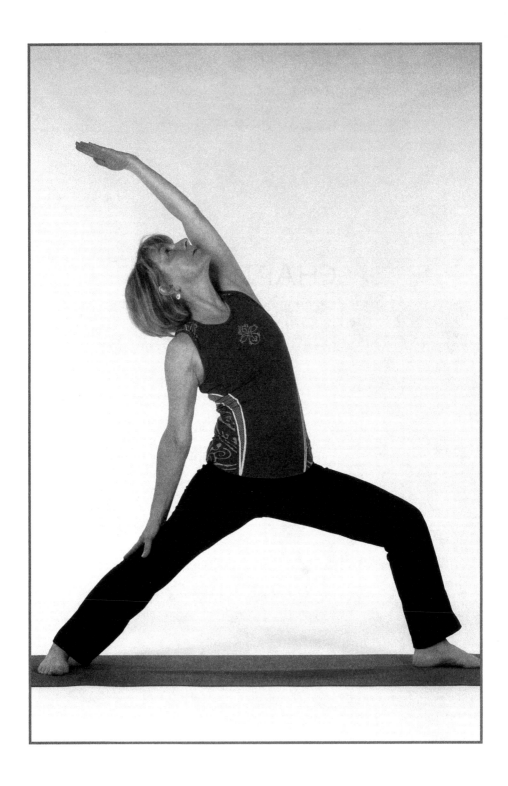

Even though an active lifestyle is healthy, there are some exercises that may actually cause more harm than good. If you have multiple sclerosis, it is best to avoid overexerting yourself with exercise or physical activity because MS symptoms become exacerbated by pushing too hard. Yoga is one beneficial practice that can be safely modified to aid people who have multiple sclerosis. It's important to remember that, as your body changes and matures, the way you practice yoga must also change. Approach your yoga practice with gentleness and acceptance of the body you have now, and allow it to work safely for you.

**Follow these guidelines to ensure safety when practicing yoga exercises for multiple sclerosis:**

• It is always recommended that you talk to your doctor before starting an exercise program. This is especially true if you know you have multiple sclerosis or impaired nerve function.
• Once you have the approval of your doctor, start the exercise program and ease into the more difficult moves. These gentle yoga exercises are intended to strengthen your body and relieve some of the symptoms associated with your multiple sclerosis, not aggravate them.
• If a pose seems too difficult or is painful in any way, try the variation pose instead.
• If you are currently using a wheelchair, try the chair variations of the poses as these have been designed specifically for individuals with restricted mobility.
• If you are new to yoga, you may find it best to start by holding the poses for only a few long, deep breaths. As you progress and feel more comfortable, you can begin to hold the poses for longer.
• Concentrate more on maintaining proper alignment while doing your yoga exercises and focus less on pushing over your limits. Recognize your limitations and respect them. Trying to surpass them may inflict unnecessary pain or risk of injury.
• Since everyone has varying degrees of flexibility and pain associated with multiple sclerosis and its symptoms, it is im-

portant not to gauge your level of difficulty against someone else's. Practice the yoga exercises to the degree that you can perform them comfortably and safely for your own body.

• While there are no specific yoga postures that must be avoided if you have MS, please use wisdom and listen to your body. If any of the yoga moves cause you pain or intensify your symptoms, stop immediately.

## Keep Your Cool

When your body becomes overheated, demyelinated nerves function less proficiently than normal. Because of this, it is important not to allow yourself to overheat while participating in any physical activity, including yoga. Your body will naturally cool itself over the course of a few hours, but you can also take a few simple steps to actively keep your cool. Keep these tips in mind:

• Resist the urge to crank the heat in the winter and keep the temperature of your house slightly cool.
• Take advantage of air conditioners in the warmer months.
• Stay away from heated pools, hot tubs, and saunas. On the other hand, taking a swim in a cool pool is a great form of exercise for multiple sclerosis patients. The water acts as a support for the body while the cool water controls overheating.

## How to Protect Against Injuries Associated with Falling

Since individuals with multiple sclerosis often suffer from problems with muscle strength, balance, and coordination, it important to practice safety precautions to help avoid unnecessary injuries.

**Here is a list of helpful reminders on how to protect against falls and reduce the risk of injuries:**

*When you are outdoors:*
• Use a cane, walker, or the arm of a loved one to lend support.
• Wear shoes with rubber soles and good traction to prevent slipping.
• Carry a shoulder bag or fanny pack to keep your hands free.
• Sprinkle salt or kitty litter on icy walkways in the winter months.
• Try to walk in the grass or around icy or wet sidewalks.

*When you are indoors:*
• Keep rooms well-lit. You may also consider installing night-lights in halls, stairways, and dimly-lit areas.
• Use a rubber bath mat in the shower or bathtub to protect against slipping.
• Install grab bars in the bathroom near the toilet, tub, and shower.
• Do not walk in slippers, stockings, or socks in the house. Instead, wear low-heeled shoes that offer more support and less slipping.
• Lay carpet runners on slippery floors. Be sure to tack them down or attach them with skid-proof backing.
• Make sure stairwells are lit and have railings on both sides. Don't forget to use them!
• Keep clutter to a minimum to avoid tripping hazards, especially on the floors and high-traffic areas.
• Store a flashlight by your bed in case you need to get up throughout the night.
• Buy a cordless phone and always keep it nearby. You won't have to rush to answer it, and it will be handy if you do fall and need to call for assistance.

## Yoga Adapted for Practice with a Wheelchair

Because MS attacks the central nervous system, many patients suffer from damage to the spinal cord. The spine in this state cannot properly support upright posture. Additionally, inflammation and injury of the myelin sheath impede the responsiveness of nerve signals, which impairs muscle coordination. As a result, many MS patients are confined to wheelchairs. Although you may feel limited by a wheelchair, you can still practice yoga!

When practicing yoga from a wheelchair, there are a few things to keep in mind. First, it is important to understand that wheelchair confinement significantly atrophies the muscles in the back and abdomen. Without the support of these core muscles, the spine slackens and begins to bend forward. This compresses the abdomen, rib cage, and lungs, which makes deep breathing nearly impossible. In turn, shallow breathing restricts the flow of oxygen and blood circulation, both of which exacerbate physical ailments and mobility. As a result, it is important to gradually strengthen these core muscles in working towards achieving the appropriate posture for these poses. The quality of your posture directly correlates with the benefits you will receive from yoga.

Before beginning any poses in your wheelchair, be sure to consult your doctor. It is also important that you have the assistance of a caregiver, especially if you are a beginner. Also, remember that yoga should stimulate your muscles, but your practice should never cause pain. If you experience pain during a pose, stop immediately.

Remember to breathe deeply while holding each pose (for breathing advice, see pages 23-25). Many of the seated poses in this book can be also practiced in a wheelchair.

**Here are some more wheelchair options for some of the other poses:**

**Forward Bend (see page 42)**
Begin by follow the directions for seated Mountain pose (see page 39). Hold onto your wheelchair just below the seat or place your hands on top of your thighs for support. As you inhale, lengthen through your spine. As you exhale, bend forward while maintaining the length in your spine. Hold this pose for three to five breaths and continue to breathe deeply.

**Warrior I (see page 44)**
With your feet directly below your knees, sit upright in your wheelchair. Do not lean on your chair's back support. Have an assistant place a chair in front of you. The seat should be facing away from you. Shift your hips to the left; slightly raise left buttocks off of seat.

Gradually draw your left leg back. Use your hand to position your left leg, if necessary. Slowly begin to drop your left knee forward, and bring your knee to the ground. Be sure to keep your left knee in line with your hip. If your knee does not reach the ground, have an assistant place a folded blanket under your knee.

Place your palms on the top of the chair. Inhale and extend through your back and ribcage. If possible, raise your arms above your head and interlock your fingers. Hold for three to five breaths. Repeat on the other side.

**Warrior II (see page 46)**
Sit forward while still remaining comfortable and maintaining balance. With your thighs separated and feet flat on the floor, bend your left knee at a 90-degree angle. Then fully straighten your right leg. On your next inhalation, bring your arms into the 'T' position. Focus your eyes on the fingertips of your left hand. Hold for five breaths. Repeat on the other side.

## Downward-Facing Dog (see page 50)

Press the back of your wheelchair against a sturdy wall. Have an assistant place a folding chair about two feet away, facing your wheelchair. You may fasten your safety belt as an extra precaution.

With your feet directly under your knees, place your hands on the seat of the folding chair. As you inhale, raise the top of your head, extending through your spine. Be sure to keep your chin parallel to the floor. Drop your shoulders downward. On the next exhale, press the chair forward to align your ears with your shoulders as you press your hips back and heels down. Continue to press your palms firmly into the seat for three to five breaths. Then return to an upright position.

This pose can also be done facing a wall by pressing your palms and forehead to the wall instead of the chair.

## Child (see page 74)

Have an assistant place a folding chair in front of your wheelchair. Be sure that the seat is facing you. Place a rolled-up mat on the seat of the chair. Then place a bolster cushion parallel to you, with one end resting on your lap and the other end resting on the seat of the chair. Add a folded blanket to rest your forehead on. Lean forward and rest your head on the blanket. No pressure should be on your nose. You can either rest your arms on the seat of the chair or try crossing them above your head. Close your eyes and relax your face and body. Maintain smooth, even breathing, and try to remain focused on your breath.

# CHAPTER 4

## THE POSES

# MOUNTAIN

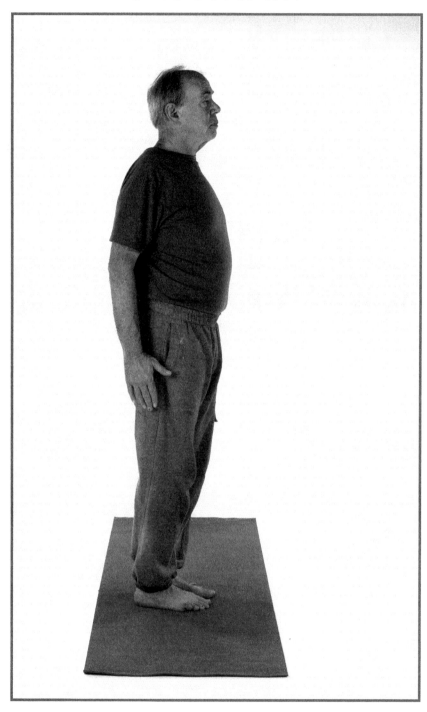

## MODIFICATION

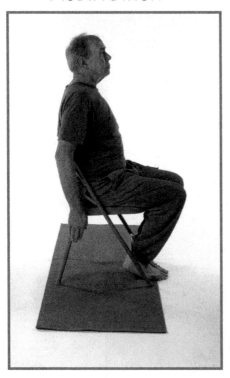

Stand with your big toes touching. Roll your shoulders up, back, and down—this movement places your shoulder blades on your back. Try to find your balance over the arches of your feet by rocking back and forth from the balls of your feet to the heels. Then build your body up from your feet and through your calves, pulling your kneecaps up, tightening your thighs, and tucking your tailbone under. Your chin should be centered with your chest. Exhale and pull up on your pelvic floor. On the next exhale, pull your stomach up and back (this will create strength in your abdominals). This "lock" in the abdominals should be used in all standing postures.

For the chair variation, sit upright in a chair with your legs and feet together and your arms at your sides. Roll your shoulders up, back, and down, then follow the directions to create a "lock" in your abdominals.

# NECK ROLLS

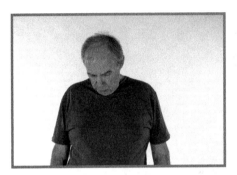
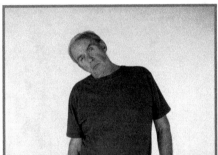
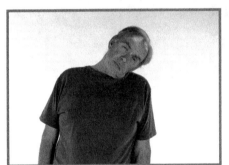
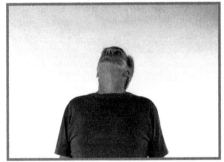

Stand with your feet together in Mountain pose (see page 38), keeping your shoulders relaxed. Roll your neck to the right, circling slowly all the way around. Go four or five times one way, then reverse and circle another four or five times in the other direction.

For the chair variation, sit upright in a chair with your back straight and feet placed on the floor. Roll your neck as stated above.

*Images are shown clockwise.*

# EAR TO SHOULDER

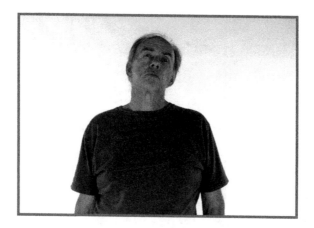

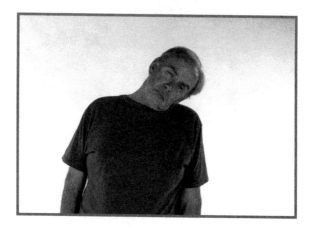

Stand with your feet together in Mountain pose (see page 38). Drop your left ear to your left shoulder and then bring your right ear to your right shoulder.

For the chair variation, sit in a chair with your back straight and feet on the floor and follow the directions above.

# WARM-UP FORWARD BEND

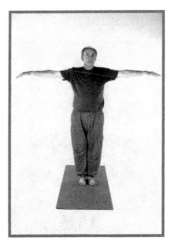

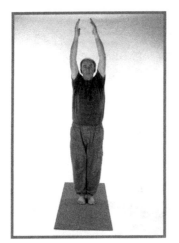

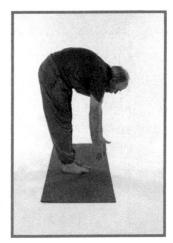

Stand with your feet together in Mountain pose (see page 38). On the inhale, sweep your arms up and over your head. Reach up and then back, stretching through both sides of your torso with your weight in your heels. On the exhale, swan-dive down into a forward bend with your arms out to your sides, leading with your chin and chest. Sweep your hands close to the floor and inhale all the way up and back again. Repeat five to six times.

## MODIFICATION

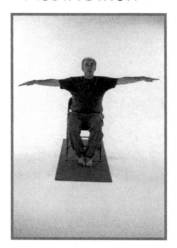

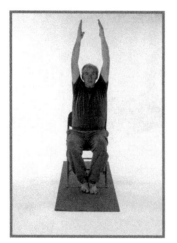
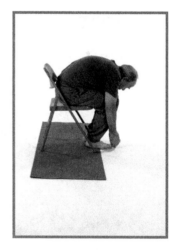

For the chair variation, sit in the chair and face forward with your legs and feet together. Sweep your arms up and then on the exhale, bend down over your legs. On the inhale, come up and reach back. In the beginning, your back may be rounded. As you gain strength, try to come down and up with a straight back.

**Note:** This pose should be done from the hips, not the waist. As always, use caution and be sure to "listen" to your body—if you feel any pain or straining in your legs or back, stop or switch to a more gentle variation.

# WARRIOR I

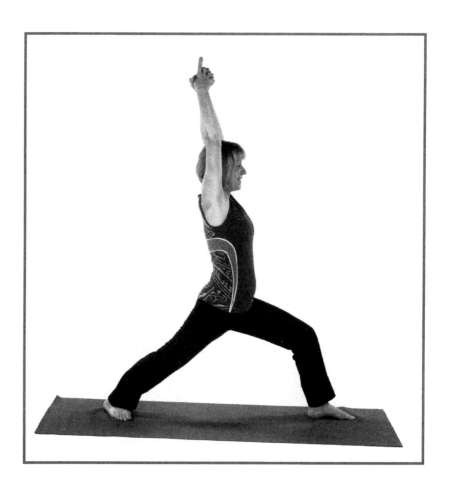

Start with your feet together in Mountain pose (see page 38). Take a wide-legged stance and turn your left foot out 90 degrees. Turn to face over your left foot with your shoulders and your hips. On the exhale, bend your left knee. On the inhale, raise your arms over your head and interlock your fingers. For increased intensity (not pictured), look up at your hands and hold for five breaths. Repeat on the other side.

MODIFICATION

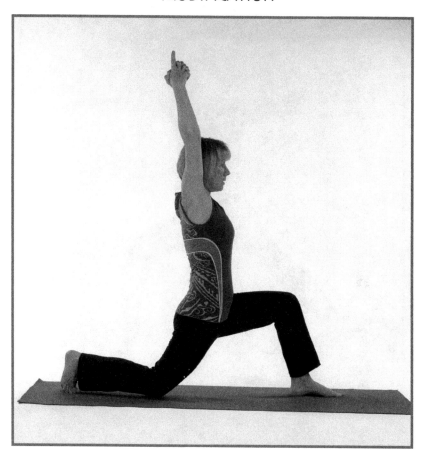

If this seems difficult, you may drop your back knee to the floor until you gain balance and strength. This may also be done with a chair: straddle the chair with your left leg bent and your right leg extended behind you, trying to turn your shoulders to the left. On the inhale, raise your arms and interlock your fingers, looking straight ahead. Once you find your balance, you may drop your head back and look up at your hands.

45

# WARRIOR II

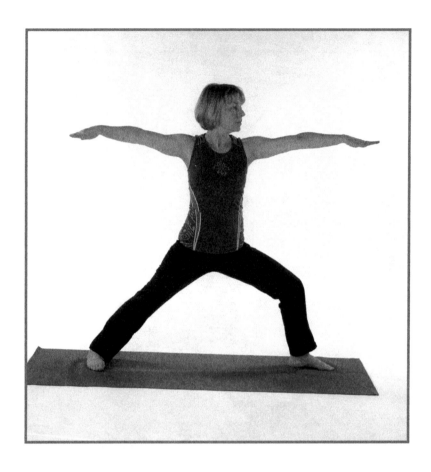

Start with your feet together in Mountain pose (see page 38).
Take a wide-legged stance and, on the exhale, turn your left
foot out 90 degrees, keeping your hips and shoulders facing
forward. On the inhale, raise your arms into a 'T' position.
On the next exhale, bend your left knee over your ankle. Your
weight should be on the outside of your right foot as you pull
up in your inner right thigh. Your focal point will be at the
fingertips of your left hand. Hold for five breaths. Repeat on
the other side.

## MODIFICATION

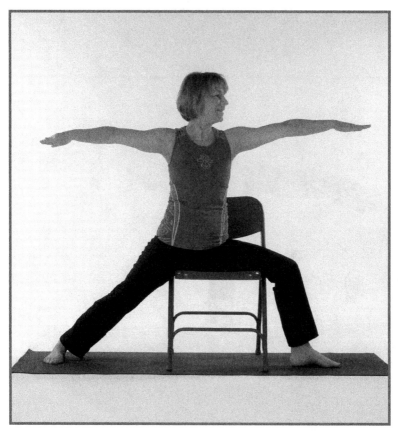

For the chair variation, sit on a chair and come to a straddle position. Bend your left knee and turn your left foot out 90 degrees. Extend your right leg out straight. On the inhale, raise your arms up and hold for five breaths.

# WARRIOR III

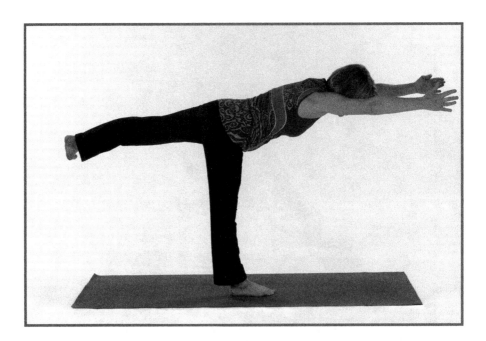

Start with your feet together, placing your weight on your right foot. On the inhale, raise your arms shoulder-width over your head. On the exhale, come forward with your torso and raise your left leg behind, keeping your hips parallel. Tighten your right leg and your abdominal muscles to hold your body up. Work up to five breaths. Repeat on the other side.

## MODIFICATION

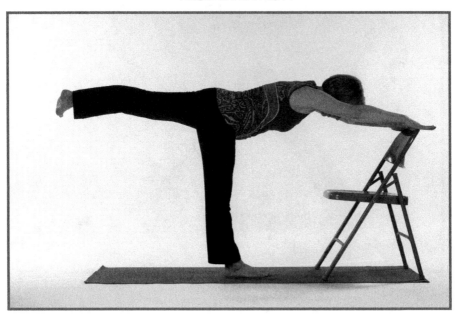

If this seems difficult, the pose can also be performed with your hands against the wall or on a chair, as shown.

**Note:** Beginners should begin by working with the chair, making sure to bend from the hips.

# DOWNWARD-FACING DOG

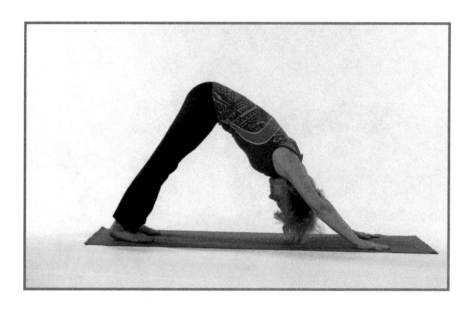

Start with your feet together in Mountain pose (see page 38).
On the inhale, raise your arms wide, up and back. On the exhale, come forward and bring your face to your knees, bending your knees as much as needed to bring your palms to the floor. On the exhale, raise your right leg and place it behind you into a runner's pose. Raise your left leg and take it back to meet the right (your feet can be together or hip-width apart). Push back through your hands and arms until you are in an inverted 'V' position. Your head should be between your arms, with your hips pushing up and heels pushing down. Your weight will be in your feet, palms, and index fingers. Hold for five breaths. To come up, step forward.

## MODIFICATION

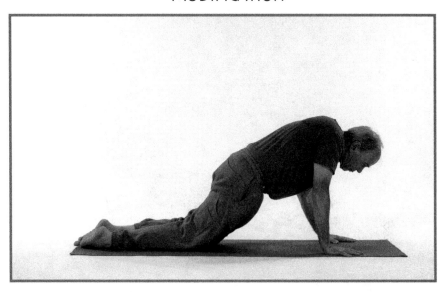

This may also be done by starting in a kneeling position on your hands and knees (in a tabletop position), then curling your toes under and pushing back into an inverted 'V' position.

# UPWARD-FACING DOG

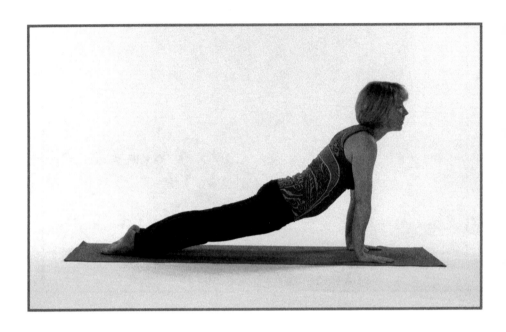

Start by lying on the mat on your stomach, with your forehead on the floor. Bring your hands under your shoulders, keeping your elbows close to your body and your legs and feet together. On the inhale, push up with your arms, raise your head, then roll your shoulders up and back, while pushing against your hands. Rising up, lift your hips and thighs off the mat so that your weight is on the top of your feet and in your hands.

## MODIFICATION

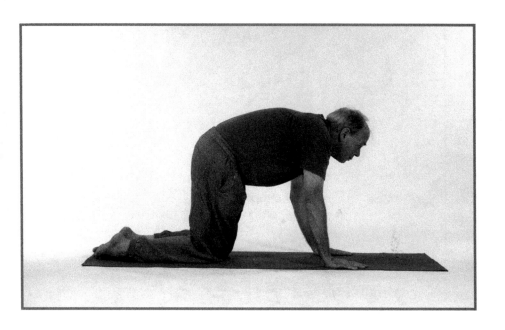

If this is difficult, you can raise up to your knees, working up to rising to your feet. Work up to five breaths.

# REVERSE WARRIOR

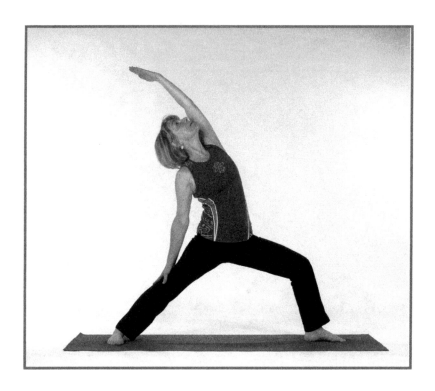

Start in Warrior II pose (see page 46), facing to the left (your
legs will not move throughout this sequence). Position your
arms out in a 'T' position. On the inhale, drop your right hand
down to your right leg as you raise your left arm straight up.
Exhale and bend your left arm over your head as you bend
your torse back, stretching the left side of your body up and
back. Hold for five breaths. Repeat on the other side.

## MODIFICATION

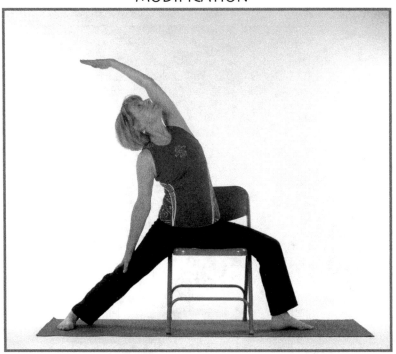

For the chair variation, start by sitting in a chair. Straddle the chair, bending your left knee as you turn your left foot out 90 degrees. Extrand your right leg out straight and then follow the arm directions.

**Note:** When moving into this back and side bend, be aware of the point where you begin to feel any resistance in the body and stop at that point. As you become more flexible, you will be able to move deeper into the pose.

# TRIANGLE

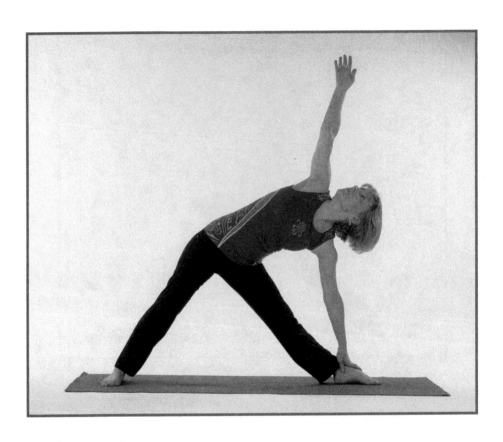

Start with your feet together in Mountain pose (see page 38) in the middle of the mat. Take a wide-legged stance and turn your right foot out 90 degrees. On the inhale, raise your arms into a 'T' position, extending them out from your shoulders. On the exhale, reach your right arm up, out, and down while pulling in on your right hip (this is a lunge movement to the right). Bring your right hand to rest on your leg wherever it goes easily (this means your hand may be as high as your knee since you are aiming for alignment of your shoulder over your leg).

## MODIFICATION

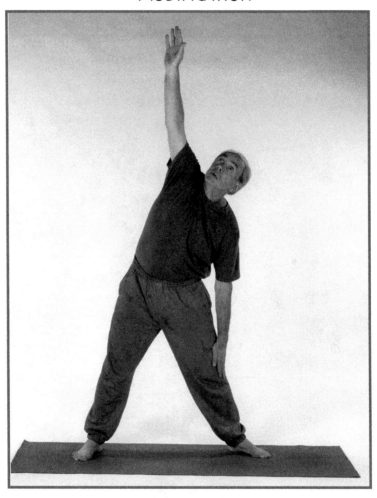

On the next breath, reach your left arm up towards the ceiling, keeping both legs straight (a block may be used here by placing it on the outside of your right foot and extending out and then down to the block). Try to turn your head to look up at your left hand; this will keep your neck in line with your spine. Hold for five breaths.

# TREE

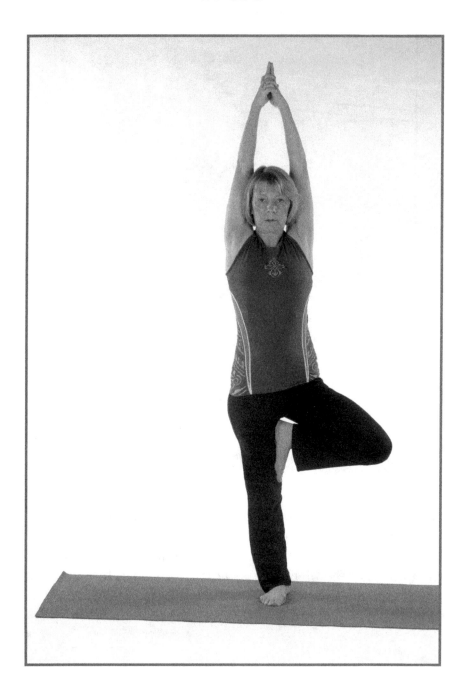

MODIFICATION 1

MODIFICATION 2

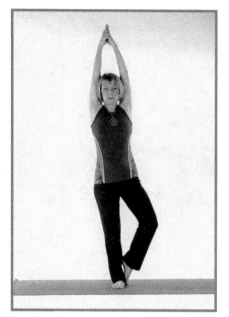

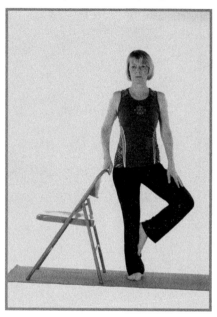

Start with your feet together in Mountain pose (see page 38). Shift your weight to your right leg and raise your left leg, placing the sole of your left foot on the inside of your right leg. Try to place your left foot as high as possible on your right leg, taking care not to place it on the inside of your knee (you may use a chair, as shown, or the wall to hold on to in the beginning). Bring your hands together in the center of your chest, with your hands in prayer position. Hold for five breaths. For increased intensity, raise your arms overhead, keeping your hands together and bringing your arms as close to your ears as possible.

# COBRA

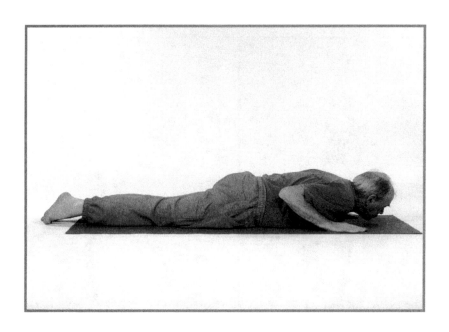

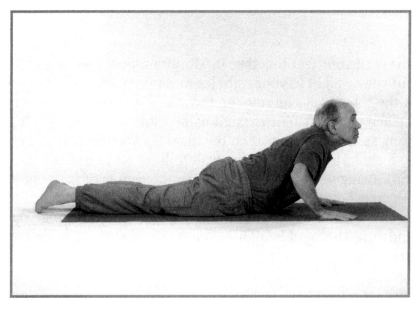

MODIFICATION

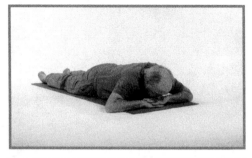

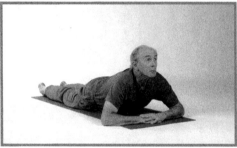

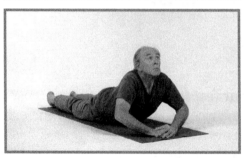

Start by lying on the mat on your stomach. Bring your feet and legs together and keep your forehead to the floor. Bring your hands under your shoulders and on the inhale, push your body up with your arms and roll your shoulders up and back while expanding your chest and keeping your hips on the floor (this will work the lower back). Hold for three full breaths and release down. Come up again and hold for three more full breaths.

**Note:** As always, use caution and be sure to "listen" to your body—if the pose becomes too difficult, stop or switch to a more gentle variation.

# PLANK

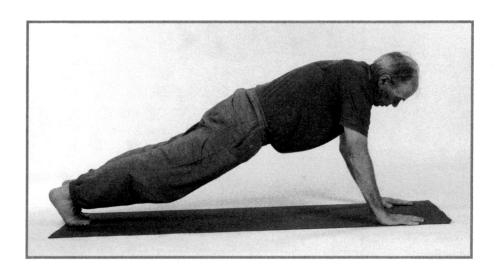

Start with your feet together in Mountain pose (see page 38). On the inhale, sweep your arms up. On the exhale, bend forward and swan-dive down. Bend your knees as needed to place your hands on the floor under your shoulders. Step your feet back and create a straight line with your body. Hold for five breaths. For increased intensity (not pictured), you may perform a side plank. Make sure your right hand is directly under your right shoulder and roll over onto the right side, trying to stack your feet one on top of the other. You can then also try to raise your left arm or keep it at your waist. Come back to the center plank and roll onto the left side (if performing the side plank).

## MODIFICATION

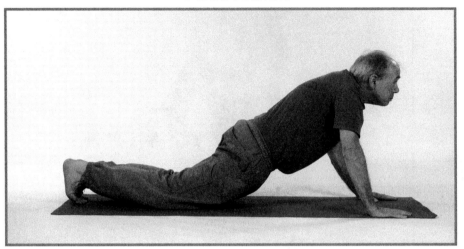

For beginners, start on your hands and knees (in a tabletop position) and step one foot back at a time until you can hold the pose with both feet back.

# BOAT

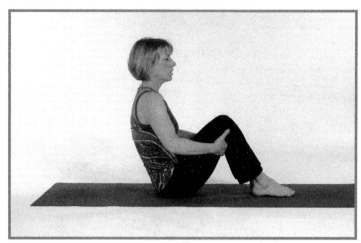

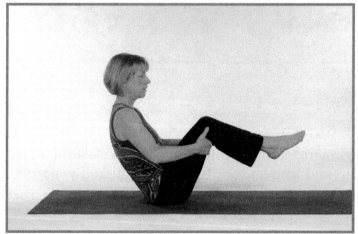

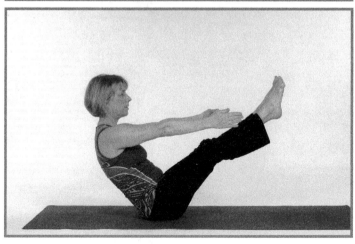

## MODIFICATION

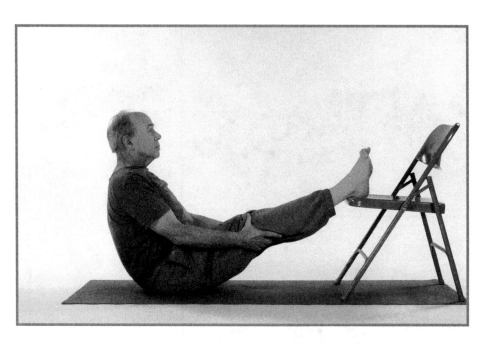

Come to a sitting staff position (sit on the mat with your back straight and your legs out in front of you). Bend your knees and bring the soles of your feet to the floor as you grab behind your knees. Rock back, holding your legs until your feet come off the floor. Try to straighten your legs and hold (you may continue to hold your legs until your abdominal muscles become strong enough to hold your body up). For increased intensity, stretch your arms out along the sides of your legs and hold for five or more breaths.

For the chair variation, place a chair in front of you and bring your feet onto the edge of the chair, proceeding as described above. If this is difficult, use a block to hold the feet up for less intensity.

# LOCUST

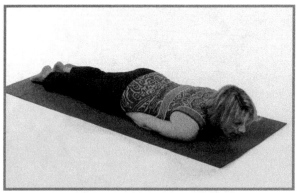

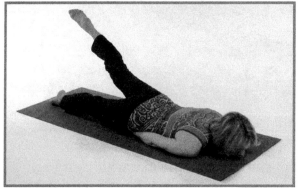

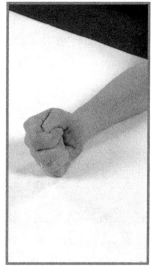

Lie on your stomach with your chin on the floor and your legs and feet together. Make a fist with your hand by wrapping your fingers around your thumbs. Bring your hands under your body at your groin. On the inhale, raise your left leg and hold for up to five breaths. Lower your leg and, on the next inhale, raise your right leg and hold, keeping your chin on the floor.

*Variation 1 (not pictured)*: Bring your hands under your body with your palms down and pinkies touching. Repeat the sequence.

## MODIFICATION

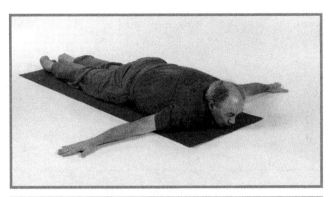

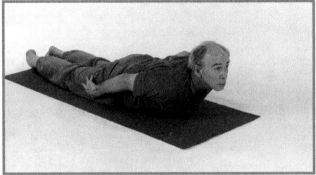

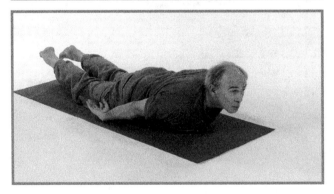

*Variation 2:* Bring your arms out in a 'T' position and, on the inhale, sweep them back and raise your head and chest. Raise your legs.

MODIFICATION

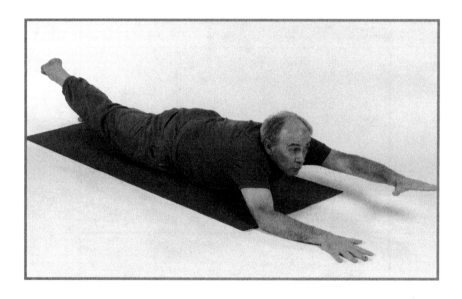

*Variation 3:* Bring your arms out in front of your body and raise your left arm and right leg, hold, then lower. Raise your right arm and left leg, hold, then lower. Finally, raise both arms and both legs (not pictured), hold, then lower.

## MODIFICATION

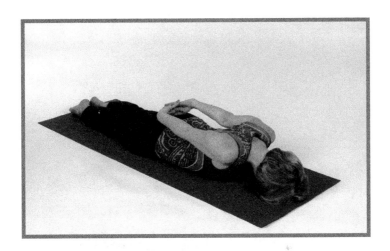

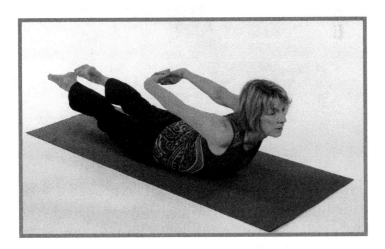

*Variation 4:* Bring your hands behind your back and interlock your fingers. On the inhale, raise your head, chest, and arms. Then raise your legs, hold, and breathe.

# REVOLVED LUNGE

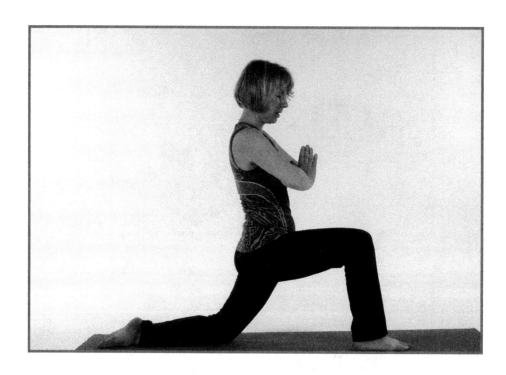

Start with your feet together in Mountain pose (see page 38).
On the inhale, sweep your arms up. On the exhale, lower into
a forward bend and place your hands on the floor. Step your
left leg back into a runners pose, bringing your body up into a
low lunge (with your back knee on the floor).

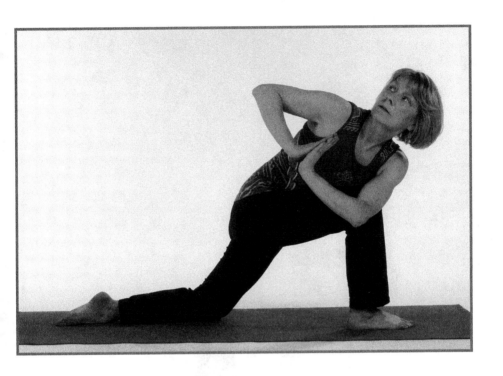

On the next inhale, raise your arms up. On the exhale, bring
your palms together and twist to the right, bringing your left
elbow to the outside of your right knee. (For a harder modification, raise your left knee off the floor before the twist).
For increased intensity (not pictured), bring your left hand to
the floor or a block and keep your right arm at your waist or
raise it and turn your head to look at your hand. (When using
the block, remember that it has three heights and beginners
should start with the highest level.)

## MODIFICATION

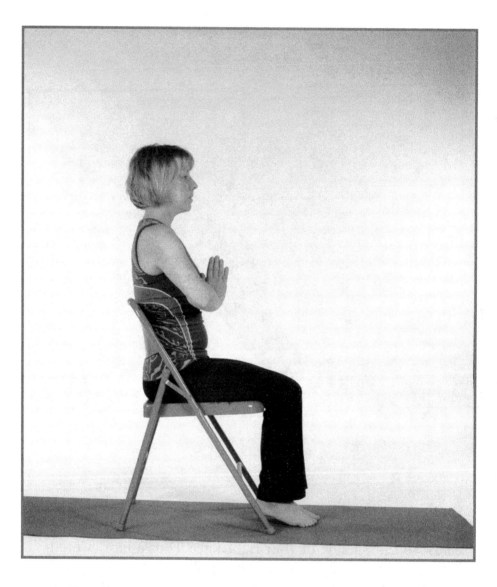

For the chair variation, sit upright in the chair with both feet placed on the floor. On the inhale, raise your arms over your head.

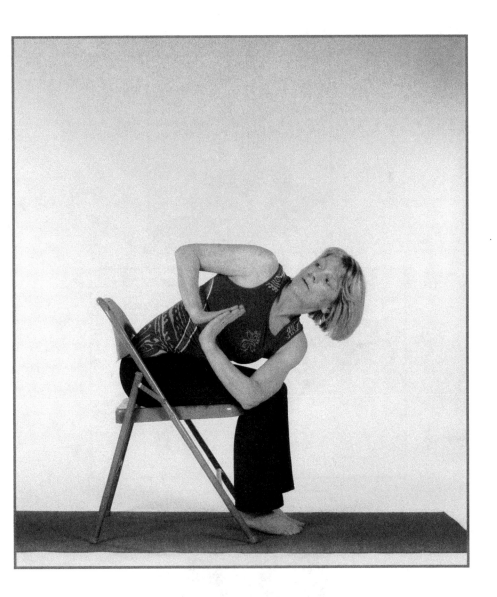

On the exhale, bring your hands together and twist to the right, trying to place the outside of your left elbow on the outside of your right knee while looking over your right shoulder. Work up to holding the pose for five breaths and then repeat on the left side.

# CHILD

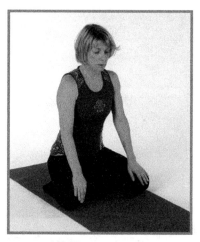

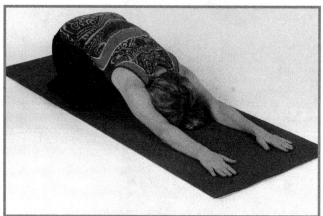

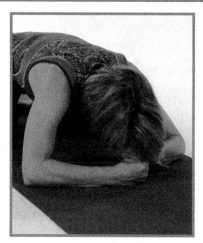

## MODIFICATION 1

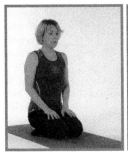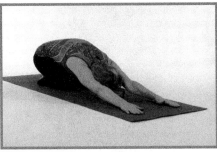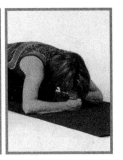

## MODIFICATION 2

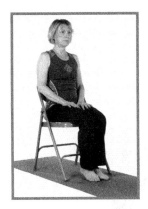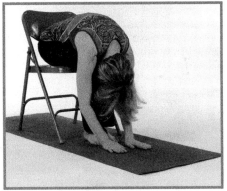

Kneel on the mat, separate your knees, and sit back on your heels (you may also keep your knees together if this is uncomfortable). Bring your body forward, trying to touch your forehead to the floor (if this is difficult, make a fist with your hands and place your forehead on your fists).

For the chair variation, sit with your legs and feet together and roll forward with your arms by your legs and your hands at your feet.

# SPHINX

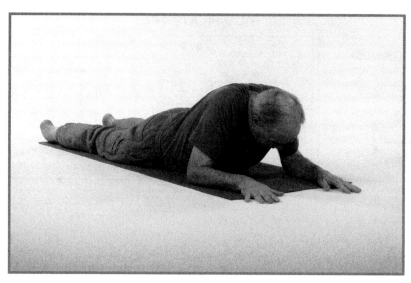

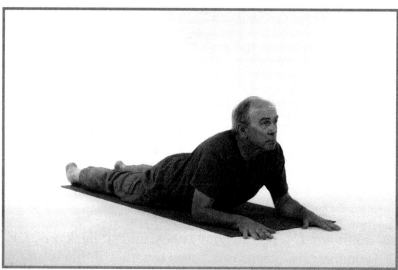

Lie on your stomach and bring your forehead to the floor. With your legs and feet together, bring your arms up and position your elbows under your shoulders, keeping your forearms stretched out in front of your torso. On the inhale, rise up onto your elbows and hold for five breaths or more. Come down, take a breath or two, and then rise back up for another five breaths.

# CORPSE

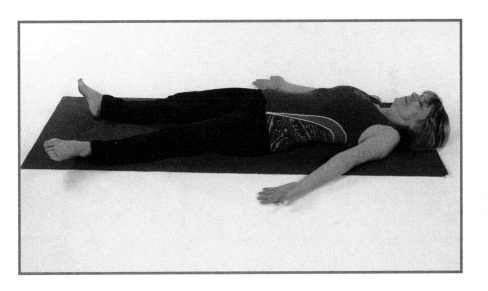

Lie on your back, with your arms extended out from your body and your palms facing up. Keep your legs a little more than hip-width apart to remove any tension from your hips. Close your eyes, bring your chin into the center of your chest, and keep your shoulders relaxed and away from your ears. Breathe deeply into your belly, letting your belly rise and fall with each breath. This pose is recommended at the end of your session to give your body a chance to relax and to allow the previous work from the poses to settle.

# CHAPTER 5

## GENTLE FLOWS FOR MULTIPLE SCLEROSIS

# STANDING LEG STRENGTH

| POSE | PAGE | EQUIPMENT |
|---|---|---|
| Mountain | 38 | chair (optional) |
| Downward-Facing Dog | 50 | |
| Triangle | 56 | block (optional) |
| Warrior I | 44 | |
| Warrior II | 46 | chair (optional) |
| Tree | 58 | chair (optional) |
| Corpse | 77 | |

# FLOOR CORE WORKOUT

| POSE | PAGE | EQUIPMENT |
| --- | --- | --- |
| Mountain | 38 | chair (optional) |
| Warm-Up Forward Bend | 42 | chair (optional) |
| Locust (4 choice variations) | 66 | |
| Boat | 64 | chair (optional) |
| Corpse | 77 | |

# FLOOR BACK, ARM, AND CORE WORKOUT

| POSE | PAGE | EQUIPMENT |
|---|---|---|
| Mountain | 38 | chair (optional) |
| Sphinx | 76 | |
| Cobra | 60 | |
| Plank | 62 | |
| Upward-Facing Dog | 52 | |
| Boat | 64 | chair (optional) |
| Child | 74 | chair (optional) |
| Corpse | 77 | |

# BALANCE

| POSE | PAGE | EQUIPMENT |
|:---:|:---:|:---:|
| Mountain | 38 | chair (optional) |
| Warm-Up Forward Bend | 42 | chair (optional) |
| Triangle | 56 | block (optional) |
| Warrior III | 48 | chair (optional) |
| Revolved Lunge | 70 | chair or block (optional) |
| Tree | 58 | chair (optional) |
| Corpse | 77 | |

# SPINE FLEXIBILITY

| POSE | PAGE | EQUIPMENT |
|---|---|---|
| Mountain | 38 | chair (optional) |
| Warm-Up Forward Bend | 42 | chair (optional) |
| Warrior II | 46 | chair (optional) |
| Reverse Warrior | 54 | chair (optional) |
| Triangle | 56 | block (optional) |
| Revolved Lunge | 70 | chair or block (optional) |
| Child | 74 | chair (optional) |
| Corpse | 77 | |

# REFERENCES

**American Yoga Association**
www.americanyogaassociation.org

**International Association of Yoga Therapists**
www.iayt.org

**Mayo Clinic**
www.mayoclinic.com

**MS Awareness Foundation**
www.msawareness.org

**Multiple Sclerosis Association of America**
www.msaa.com

**Multiple Sclerosis Foundation**
www.msfacts.org

**Multiple Sclerosis International Federation**
www.msif.org

**National Multiple Sclerosis Society**
www.nationalmssociety.org

**PubMed Health, by the U.S. National Library of Medicine (NLM)**
www.ncbi.nlm.nih.gov/pubmedhealth

**The Yoga Site**
www.yogasite.com

**Yoga Journal**
www.yogajournal.com

# LAURIE SANFORD

Laurie Sanford has practiced yoga for 14 years and is certified under Rob Greenberg, owner of the Yoga for Peace Studio in Margaretville, NY. She has been teaching for eight years and currently provides yoga instruction to adults. Laurie has trained at the Kripalu Center for Yoga and Health, as well as the Himalayan Institute. She currently resides with her husband and daughter in the Catskill Mountains, where they run a weekly newspaper.

# JO BRIELYN

Jo Brielyn is a freelance writer and author. She is a contributing writer for Hatherleigh Press and has published works in several print and online publications. Jo also owns and maintains the Creative Kids Ideas (www.creativekidsideas.com) and Good for Your Health (www.good-for-your-health.com) websites. For more information about Jo's upcoming projects or to contact her, visit www.JoBrielyn.com. Jo resides in Central Florida with her husband and two daughters.

# Check Out These Other Titles from Hatherleigh Press!

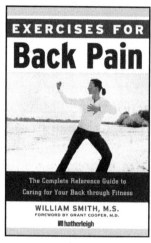

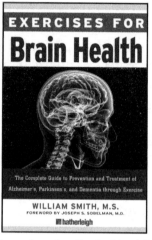

Exercises for Back Pain
ISBN 978-1-57826-304-2

Exercises for Brain Health
ISBN 978-1-57826-316-5

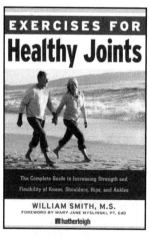

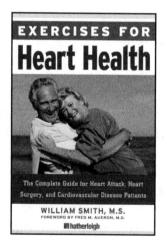

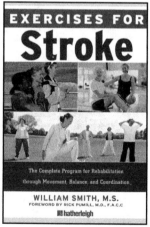

Exercises for
Healthy Joints
ISBN 978-1-57826-344-8

Exercises for Heart Health
ISBN 978-1-57826-303-5

Exercises for Stroke
ISBN 978-1-57826-317-2

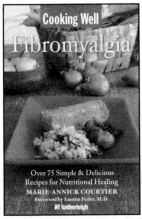
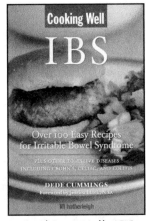

Cooking Well: Fibromyalgia
ISBN 978-1-57826-362-2

Cooking Well: IBS
ISBN 978-1-57826-388-2

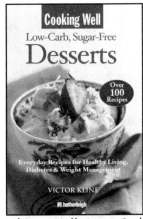
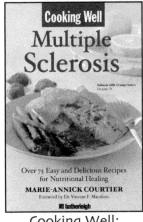
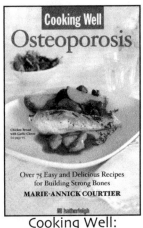

Cooking Well: Low-Carb
Sugar-Free Desserts
ISBN 978-1-57826-325-7

Cooking Well:
Multiple Sclerosis
ISBN 978-1-57826-301-1

Cooking Well:
Osteoporosis
ISBN 978-1-57826-302-8

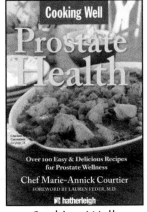
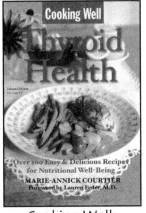
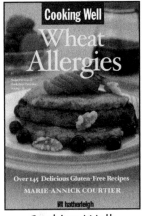

Cooking Well:
Prostate Health
ISBN 978-1-57826-376-9

Cooking Well:
Thyroid Health
ISBN 978-1-57826-352-3

Cooking Well:
Wheat Allergies
ISBN 978-1-57826-313-4

# Also in the Gentle Yoga Series

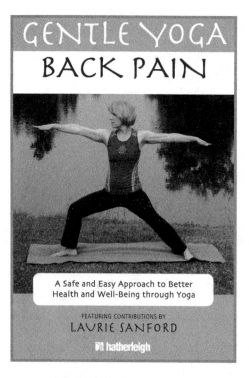

Gentle Yoga for Back Pain
ISBN 978-1-57826-390-5

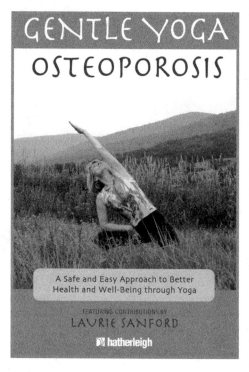

Gentle Yoga for Osteoporosis
ISBN 978-1-57826-397-4

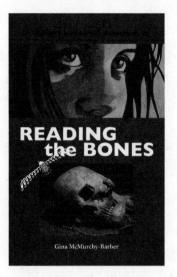
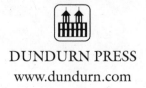

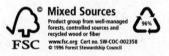
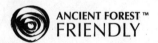